Journey to the

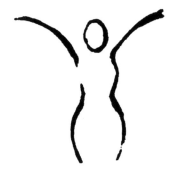

Shape of You

*A Seven Week Course in
Discovering and Recovering
Your Ideal Weight Through the
Pathway of Journaling*

Marian Willingham

Journey to the Shape of You

Library of Congress Control Number: 00-91987

Cover: Cheryl Stacy & Jill Knight

ISBN: 0-9700954-0-6

Published by Backwater Publishing
241 N. Washington, Cloverdale, CA 95424

Printed in the USA by Morris Publishing
3212 E. Hwy. 30, Kearney, NE 68847

I would like to dedicate this book to all of the clients I have had the privilege of working with in my business, **The Shape of You.**
The inspiration for this book came from
the many people who have
shown the courage to finally heal their
relationship with food . . . forever.

ACKNOWLEDGMENTS

I wish to acknowledge my two best friends
and wonderful typesetters
Jill Knight and Cheryl Stacy,
and the most knowledgeable
and patient peer-reader Sarah Spinner,
also the two sweetest dogs a woman could
ever own, Libby and Max, whose constant
companionship made the long hours of this
journey so much more enjoyable.

CONTENTS

INTRODUCTION

"MARIAN YOU ARE ON THE CUSP OF SOARING..."

I will never forget those words spoken to me by a special someone who knew I was in the middle of a significant and powerful life change. The change was my final release from dysfunction with food. Previously I had thought, how can I soar when I have these chains around my ankles? The chains were my total obsession with food and losing weight. Even when I lost weight I was not satisfied. I still felt fat at 10 pounds under my ideal weight. My problem was, I did not love myself at any weight. How then could I ever be satisfied with any results?

My internal and external struggles with my body, as well as my addiction to food, began in fifth grade. I remember the day I stayed home from school and ate a whole box of chocolate cupcakes in 3 hours. I did not want them. I was not physically hungry. I was emotionally hungry, a type of hunger I would understand more about years later. I was sad. I did not want to go to school and stand in the free lunch ticket line again, only to be teased and humiliated by the kids in the regular line.

I hated my new school and my intense loneliness created a new level of emotional hunger.

For years I tried to satisfy emotional hunger with food. As the numbers on the scale rose, family members noticed and commented on my increasing body size. These comments made me feel ashamed of my weight, which only lowered my already low self-esteem and my overall lack of self-worth.

I discovered the sacred skill of sneak eating. When I turned 16, I was so happy to have the privacy of my car to escape and over-indulge in food. I knew the menu at every drive-through by heart. Still, I could not seem to satisfy my intense emotional hunger. No food seemed to satisfy the profound sense of emptiness.

In my 20's I became an expert at the game of losing and regaining weight. Losing weight, however, became my true forté. I used laxatives, spent 2 years of my life addicted to prescription diet pills, and then discovered the ultimate release of food and all this built up emotion: bulimia. All of these endeavors made sense to me at the time but I remained trapped in a tiny world that revolved solely around my body and the food I put in and took out of it. It wasn't until my husband was diagnosed with leukemia that I could no longer control my poisonous relationship with food. The rug was being pulled out from underneath me and I was falling. As I was dealt the hand of a caregiver, my weight and obsession with food skyrocketed. I was overcome by my fear of the future and the loss of my life as I had known it to be.

One day during my husband's treatment, I took a walk and came upon a beautiful pink stucco Spanish-styled building at the base of the San Gabriel mountains. A sign on the building read, "WOMAN'S HEALING CENTER."

The words themselves comforted me. I wanted to go into the inviting entrance and check myself in. More than anything in my life I wanted to be healed...but healed from what?

I was not able to label my pain. I felt completely alone, overwhelmed about my secret dysfunction with food.

And so now I offer you the kind of validation I needed then. This book not only allows you to accept and understand your own dysfunction, but will give you the tools to heal it as well. I am grateful that I saw that sign. It comforted me. It touched me in a way that encouraged me to heal. I will always remember the sense of inner peace the words "WOMAN'S HEALING CENTER" brought me. I knew that one day I would create my own sort of woman's healing center. I did, and now I have the words that offer other women a sense of safety and a fresh starting point for their process toward full recovery from eating-related issues.

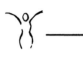

WHY I WROTE THIS BOOK

I spent my thirtieth year healing my relationship with food. I began to realize and eventually internalize the fact that there are 3 types of hunger: physical, emotional and spiritual. Unfortunately, many of us eat from all three. To heal our relationship with food, we must understand why we suffer from emotional and spiritual hunger. It's not what we are eating that creates the problems we have with food; it is what is eating at us.

I spent an entire year learning about how I developed such a painful and desperate relationship with food. I healed myself and healed the pain of the past. I also lost weight. Since that time I have been my ideal weight. I eat whatever I want when I am PHYSICALLY hungry, and I have never felt more whole, more at peace, more grateful to be alive in this body.

There are many great books on the subject of recovery from dysfunctional eating. Many encourage readers to eat what you crave, eat when you are physically hungry, and stop when you are satisfied. But I believe that we must first heal the wounds that lead us to the overwhelming emotional and spiritual hungers that plague us before we can follow these guidelines. Purchasing the book is easy, practically applying the principals into one's everyday life is hard. That is where I come in. I take my clients through the process of applying the steps into a daily routine, one that can eventually become second nature.

After recovering from compulsive overeating, I was inspired to leave my 15 year career as a hairdresser and become a personal eating coach. I found it unfulfilling to make a person feel beautiful from the outside in, as this only lasts temporarily. I wanted to help them feel beautiful from the inside out to support the kind of change that lasts forever.

My business THE SHAPE OF YOU has grown rapidly. This book is everything I teach to my clients. In the past 3 years I have worked with doctors, lawyers, bus drivers, college professors, mothers, artists...anyone interested in living a life without food and weight obsession. While using the techniques that evolved from my practice, I have seen lives transformed. Clients are empowered by discovering the underlying issues that caused years of dysfunction with food.

I began to recognize the common problems all of my clients seemed to have and the roadblocks that they all had to move through to be successful in this process. I recognized these roadblocks because they were my roadblocks too.

I will never forget a desperate phone call I received one day from a new client who wanted to work with me to lose the 40 pounds she had gained during the 3 years she had been married. She called in a panic, absolutely horrified to learn that her husband had purchased tickets to the Virgin Islands without her knowledge. She had avoided planning for a vacation because she was terrified to wear a bathing suit and reveal her body in public. Most of us know the pain and fear that accompanies this dilemma.

This woman was living in her husband's sweat pants and large shirts in order to hide the fact that she had gained the weight (of course he probably noticed anyway.) I told her that my work did not produce the 20-pounds-off-in-6-weeks results. My program was not about a diet; it was about a change in attitude and awareness .

We could not just put a Band-aid on the problem. Her problem was this: compulsively turning to food and gaining weight. We would work together to understand how she became a compulsive overeater and then heal her relationship with food.

She agreed to work with me. As we began the process of unraveling her fears, I encouraged her to go to the store and purchase some cute clothes for her vacation. She was reluctant to do so as she dreaded seeing her reflection in the department store mirror. She did not want to face her image. I tried to help her understand that she deserved to buy pretty new clothes no matter what size she was. She was still a beautiful person inside, I told her, and she needed to nurture that side of herself.

She went to a discount store because she felt totally revolted by her physical appearance and did not feel worthy of commercial department store prices. She tried on bathing suits and shorts and as she predicted, felt traumatized by the reality of her body size. She raced home and as soon as her husband went to bed she ate everything she could get her hands on. The very thing that betrayed her, food, was the very thing she turned to for comfort.

Eventually, she went to the mall and bought some fun vacation clothes. On her trip she discovered over conversations with other women that she had experienced something quite common. Most of the women she met had gone through the same packing issues in preparation for their trips. Her struggle is indeed a common one and one that can be extinguished...slowly.

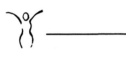

THIS CAN WORK FOR YOU

The pathway of recovery from compulsive overeating is an emotional detoxification process. We must bring out negative beliefs about ourselves and our self-worth, experience them, understand them and let them go. There is no easy way to heal our obsession with food or our distorted self-perceptions. There is no map that tells us where to go. Instead, there is only a learn-as-you-go process, one I will assist you with, that will lead you along your own path toward healing and recovery. There is no perfect set of rules or list of rights and wrongs that applies to everyone. Healing your obsession with food requires listening to yourself and honoring your unique experience.

As I have kept track of the consistent cycles of growth my clients go through I have realized that this could be a book. Just think about the possibilities of eating all of your favorite foods while reaching and maintaining an ideal weight forever. Imagine being totally released from yo-yo dieting, deprivation, and the inevitable weight regain. Through the exercises in this book, you will begin a journey of finding out why you have carried the burden of overeating.

I know these steps work. Before working with me, my clients have struggled with numerous diets only to lose and then regain weight, often finding themselves heavier than when they began their diets. I believe in this process. My clients have demonstrated so much courage in their own healing. I'm inspired every time I see someone understand for the first time what is actually eating at them. And guess what? It just might be the most frightening experience of your life to finally realize what is actually eating at you.

In order to heal our relationship with food we must first turn around and face our dysfunction with food, embrace it,

9

forgive it and finally let it go. We cannot go back; we can only move forward on a positive pathway. Regardless of age, lifestyle or personal problems, it is not too late to heal this affliction.

If you are a compulsive overeater then you are a person who turns to food for comfort. After doing so, you shamed yourself with self-judgement. You might be used to this negative self-talk cycle. Your need to use food as comfort is about to end. You are about to learn the truth: YOU are the only one who can truly comfort YOU.

Now is the beginning of your own journey along the pathway to the shape of you.

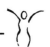

THE PATHWAY
TO HEALING

pathway (path•way) *a path, course; a sequence of reactions.*

healing (he`ling) *growing sound.*

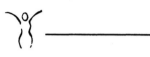

THE JOURNAL

Why journal? As we begin the process of healing our relationship with food, we begin uncovering the underlying reasons we began to use food to help cope with the pain and difficulties life presented. IT'S NOT WHAT WE ARE EATING, IT IS WHAT IS EATING AT US.

It becomes clear that our deeper problems and needs must be dealt with. Believe it or not, food is not the issue. Developing a balance between the inner and outer self sheds light on the areas in our lives that need attention, thus enabling us to make changes with our approach toward food and eating. This will eventually lead to a healthy change in our weight. We reveal the areas in our lives where we need to make changes with food and our weight. Journal writing encourages internal balance as we look within, where all the answers reside.

By journaling your way through the seven weekly assignments, you will devise your own routine for getting much needed inner nourishment and it will become a daily practice, and eventually a natural way of life.

Whenever I suggest the journal process to clients, they often want to know how to do this. Journal writing is done by you and for you. There is no right or wrong way to keep a journal.

Clients often express that they are afraid to journal because of the pain they know they will uncover. Sometimes they are actually afraid of what might appear on the page. My usual response is to remind them of how good it will feel to release all of the bad thoughts and feelings and to imagine how good it will feel to let all of this pain go.

Pretend that all the pain of the past we keep stored in our minds is a beach ball. Imagine yourself in the deep end of a swimming pool holding the beach ball under water. After awhile your arms get tired and you realize that you can no longer hold onto the ball. You are afraid to let go of the ball though, because you have no control over where it will land. The landing of the ball will change all the dynamics in your life. Such is the powerful experience of journaling as an aid toward healing.

It is okay to be afraid. One of the most powerful lessons to be learned during the recovery process is that **the opposite of fear is trust.** Now is the time to turn that fear around and begin to trust.

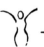

OUR HEALING PATHWAY

We have all the answers inside of us. Our wisdom resides within us. We need to re-connect to our inner trust. By doing this we can re-connect to what it means to be hungry and what we are hungry for. Freeing yourself from a weight problem means learning to trust the body and its cravings.

As you begin to trust your body's cravings and re-connect to your inner voice of physical hunger, something profound will take place. You will begin to not only understand but actually experience the difference between **physical, emotional and spiritual hungers.** When you ask yourself, "am I hungry and what am I hungry for?" your inner voice might respond with being hungry for a nap or maybe a hug from a close friend. Not food. These are the things you will learn along the way during the journey through the steps in this book.

I designed the book to be a seven week journal workbook. That way, as you work on each week it will ground you in the truth of each step. When I first start working with clients they are usually afraid **(fear)** to believe **(trust)** that this philosophy can actually work, that the very thing that has turned against them might become a pleasurable experience. I assure them that the eating experience is supposed to be pleasurable.

As we work together, I see the client dare to dip a toe into the pond of truth, as the weeks roll by I begin to see the client go from dipping a toe to wading knee deep. After pausing to give the experience some time and reflection, clients begin to lose weight as they submerge themselves into the pond and swim with complete trust in themselves. Their bodies release weight while they eat foods they love and honor spiritual and emotional hungers appropriately.

It is hard to make a commitment to lose weight *and* work on the reasons we have decided to satisfy our emotional and spiritual hungers with food, but the two go hand in hand. Journal writing helps us along as it increases self-understanding and self-esteem. It furthers growth. We all want self-love, inner peace and a strong sense of self. Through journal writing we explore the inner truths without shame. Our thoughts can become a channel toward growth, a growth unconcerned with logic or consistency.

STARTING A JOURNAL

The initial decision to start a journal is yours. In today's rat-race society we get caught up in fulfilling so many external obligations that we end up neglecting our own needs. The resentment builds and we are left with a feeling of unhappiness and emptiness.

Start with the belief that you are worthy of 20 minutes a day of quiet time to write. All the potential benefits of keeping a journal are yours. Journaling to heal your spirit is certainly worth 20 minutes a day. How can we make our garden blossom if we do not take the time to water and care for it? This contact with the inner self is an imperative prerequisite to a happy and healthy existence.

With every exercise in the book, look at yourself coming into a room through someone else's eyes. Come into that room with total awareness, with strong boundaries knowing that you have the choice to say no to people, to rise above negativity, to avoid blaming others, to have a strong sense of self, believing that you deserve.

If you consistently work through the following exercises, a breakthrough will follow. When we diet we only put a Band-Aid on the problem. When we work through what is eating at us we come away from the experience healed and able to have a healthy relationship with food.

As we begin the process of healing our relationship with food, we begin to uncover the real reasons we use food to help deal with our emotions, loneliness, anxiety, and depression. Regaining balance in your life will help you let go of food issues forever.

You will discover unlimited potential. Surely all of these rewards are worth 20 minutes of writing a day. This book is about your own writing. You will be guided through the seven steps that help to release you from food obsession and compulsive overeating.

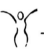

WHEN TO JOURNAL

I feel the best time to journal is right before you fall asleep. If you can develop a routine of working through the steps in your journal while sitting in bed then it will get done. We are all so busy from the time we rise until the time we go to bed. When we establish that special quiet time at night, we find a comfortable space, mental and physical, in which to sit, reflect and write.

I promise that you will start to look forward to this time. It is for **you.** I also encourage you to carry your journal with you throughout the day. As you begin working the seven steps, you will have new insights to your reaction to food. You will also become aware of the best times for you to eat. It will vary day to day because physical hunger is erratic.

These assignments are not to be graded or judged. They do not need to make sense or seem creative. This is your unique expression of healing.

RE-CONNECTING TO SELF

Journal writing is the key to understanding how you got so disconnected with true physical hunger. In the beginning make 20 minutes of writing a day your goal. You might become addicted to the page and the sky will be the limit to your private journal time.

Tapping into your new relationship with food happens in three stages. First we acknowledge that we often eat when we are not physically hungry. Before beginning the healing process we may have denied this. Maybe you devour a whole meal's worth of food while preparing dinner, for example, because you are not totally aware that you are doing it. The second stage consists of being aware of *when* we are eating. We also become aware of *what is eating at us*. This awareness leads to the commitment to a new approach. The third stage produces two results from this empowering process; weight loss and a greater sense of self. We begin to honor our feelings instead of burying them under a box of chocolates.

Recording this experience in a journal not only validates you, it enlightens you. An understanding of your strengths and weaknesses can emerge

As you may know, denial is a stage in which we do not even know we have a problem. When people go on a "diet" they are told what to eat and when. They cling to a false sense of control while struggling with the inner critical voice who enforces strict rules. In this program, when you heal your relationship with food, you become aware that you were blindly eating to avoid assuming responsibility for eating or overeating something that gave you feelings of remorse or guilt. When you are in denial about eating without awareness, it is easy to place the blame elsewhere.

Some clients tell me they cannot understand why they are overweight because they hardly ever eat. They might blame it on a slow thyroid, a slow metabolism or even on a mysterious genetic problem. Yes, people can be clinically diagnosed with these conditions, but most likely, these clients are in total denial about how much food they are consuming during the day. It is easier to focus on the outside of themselves as opposed to the unknown issues within. It is scary to grow, to heal. Numbing oneself with food is, at times, a comforting alternative to feeling true feelings, to experiencing and ultimately resolving inner conflicts.

THE THREE HUNGERS

When we think about hunger and what it means to be physically hungry, most of us think about the sensation of being ravenous, being hungry to the point of starving. *Physical hunger* is about 10 to 20 minutes from that point. Journal writing will allow you to become aware of your response to the three hungers. Your reasons for eating when not physically hungry, or overeating, or both, will become clear. *Emotional hunger,* on the other hand, is defined as anxiety, boredom, not being able to sleep etc. *Spiritual hunger* is often more difficult to acknowledge. It often appears as the feeling of a void or lack of excitement about one's place in life, the need to find inner peace, etc. Through journaling, you will discover how often you eat in response to all three hungers.

Spending time in solitude with your journal signifies self-nurturing. It will give you insight into how you became so dysfunctional with food and out of control with your weight.

It is normal to resist the journal. I tell my clients this; *the thing we resist the most in life is the very thing that keeps us from our dreams.* The "thing" we are resisting may be difficult to identify, but I assure you that these exercises will help you to explore your hidden obstacles.

If you do not feel like doing the journal writing, you may want to write this statement down and post it in a place where you will read it a couple of times a day.

Good luck and prepare yourself for a very exciting seven weeks.

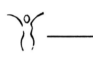

PART 1

WEEK 1

THE PATHWAY TO HEALING:

AWARENESS

AWARE (a•ware)
mindful.

Relearning awareness is the beginning of your **Journey to the Shape of You.** The first weekly assignment: healing a lack of awareness in your life.

The first step to healing a lack of awareness in your life and making changes in your relationship with food is *learning to be in a state of awareness.* This involves paying attention to **where** you are and **who** you are in that moment. A positive outcome of such awareness is that you will learn to sustain those feel-good moments, those sensations of inner relaxation with regard to food and eating. You will get as much enjoyment out of life and eating as you can. Why live a life without the genuine light of self-awareness?

Part of becoming aware requires noting your discomfort, even honoring it. Most people resort to numbing their uncomfortable feelings with food. Unfortunately, many of us have allowed fear of discomfort to block our awareness. I have found this to be true over and over again with clients and before that, with myself. We would rather remain unaware than find out why the discomfort exists.

A letter I received from a client perfectly exemplifies this awareness avoidance:

"...just ran out of diet pills I was taking and have now switched to another brand which probably won't do anything at all...I know you don't favor this approach but at least it gives me an added emotional edge...Sunday I just mostly ate protein bars to get rid of hunger without wanting to do any real eating. Monday I was so hungry. Could this be due to the diet pills? Anyway I was having a hard day emotionally. I spent the morning paying bills and trying to balance my checkbook, which is very draining for me. Then I started to think about my future and the fact that I would like to be in a relationship. Thoughts like this send me over the edge. I wonder why I am so terrified of meeting someone new. Maybe I am terrified of not being liked, or terrified of getting into a relationship that will eventually break up. I can't bear the thought of going through another break up. I'm also terrified of being too fat for someone, not to mention too old.

I wound up eating an ice cream bar in the afternoon yesterday which tasted so good and I have to admit, made me feel a lot better. I rationalized that I probably wouldn't want much else during the day and I didn't until I ate a big chocolate chip cookie. Ok, I thought, still no great damage and it was around 6:00pm so I figured I was in the clear. But by 10:00pm I was hungry again and ate a can of salmon...which I had to share with my cat. Then I had some frozen yogurt and cereal with chocolate sauce. Not a lot actually. It felt like the right amount of food and then I was done but I didn't feel like I had been in a state of awareness for the day..."

My client's avoidance of awareness due to her discomfort comes through in her writing. What was really going on? It seems her fear of meeting someone new and her financial stress have contributed to some anxiety, that has made her run to food for comfort. A preoccupation with her eating in general allows her to avoid feeling real pain.

The awareness exercises paid off. She began to eat what she really wanted in a state of awareness. The weight loss was her happy reward. But it was hard for her to get to that place of awareness as she was under the spell of diet pills, the threat of a new relationship and the financial pressure of various bills.

When we are completely aware of all that is going on, we are able to take stock in ourselves and trust in the strength of our inner resources. Why put limitations on ourselves by going through life unaware of what we are feeling and experiencing moment to moment? In the state of awareness with food, we are able to enjoy what we choose to eat while we eat it.

If, for example, we give ourselves permission to eat cupcakes and we sit down with a plate of four cupcakes in front of the television we will probably overeat. We will eat past satisfaction, all four cupcakes and not even enjoy the taste. We are left with a sensation of being full.

If, however, we sit down with a plate of four cupcakes and eat them in complete awareness, we will probably eat only one or two. Our awareness will allow us to experience the sensation of fullness. In that awareness, we are able to have the pleasure of the food without the discomfort of overeating. **The only reward for overeating is weight gain.**

The first assignment I give to new clients to teach them about this kind of awareness is; go to the grocery store, purchase all of their favorite and previously forbidden foods. I explain that they can eat the foods as long as they do it in complete awareness.

I gave this assignment to a very special client, "Gloria." She shared with me in our next session that she purchased many cans of condensed milk. She said that she was obsessed with the creamy milk and usually only had it around during the holiday season for baking. I asked her why she chose the condensed milk when she could get any goodies at the store. She told me that she loved the taste of the milk by itself.

After working with me for a few months, Gloria began to eat in complete awareness. She realized that it was not the taste of the canned milk she was after but the feeling associated with a particular memory. When she was a small girl in Cuba, before the Castro regime, her mother used to regularly cook with the condensed milk. The smell and taste reminded her of her mother. As the youngest of six children, Gloria spent many hours with her mother in the kitchen, watching her mother prepare the family meals.

Gloria's mother died when she was a young girl, shortly after her family fled to America. The milk obsession was not about the enjoyment of the taste; it was about the memory and the emotional connection to her mother. Gloria had lost her mother prematurely and needed the memory connection.

Interestingly enough, after this discovery, Gloria found that she no longer had the desire to sample the milk. This sort of experience happens to many of my clients. When they heal deprivation from the foods they "thought" they were attracted to, they actually discover that the obsession is an illusion. There is often an important connection to the food.

When we go through our daily routine without awareness, we cheat ourselves out of the beauty and pleasure of life. How many people drive to work every day and cannot remember the drive? Usually we are completely unaware of the car moving. Auto pilot takes over and we miss the experience of the drive completely. Unfortunately for many of us, it is the same with eating.

We must become aware in order to heal compulsive overeating and food obsession. An exercise like going to the grocery store and buying favorite foods requires letting go of the diet mentality we have absorbed. We must remember that the opposite of fear is trust and we need to begin right now to trust that we are going to become aware in our life, to find the foods we truly like, and to want to eat them because they give us pleasure, not because they offer an escape from pain.

Here's a scenario I like to share with clients that exemplifies the power of the forbidden food:

When you take a group of children and in their home surround them with bowls of candy in every room, then the candy, being so readily available loses its thrill. If you take another group of children and tell them that candy is bad and that they can only have carrot sticks for a treat, you can count on this group becoming obsessed with candy.

If these two groups of children go to a birthday party where there are bowls of candy everywhere, the group that has an abundance of candy in their homes will not think anything of it. They might have a handful of the candy or they might not. But the group of children that never get the treats are going to eat them until they feel sick. They know that when they return home they will be deprived of such tasty foods.

The assignment of surrounding yourself with the favorite foods will allow you to see foods as emotionally neutral. After awhile your body will learn to make positive choices and you will re-connect to the foods that make you feel good.

We all have the experience of going on a vacation and over indulging in rich foods. If you learn to listen to your body, on returning home from vacation, you will hear your body signal to you food choices that will be far different from the rich foods you were enjoying on your trip. That is how the body will balance itself out and let go of any extra weight you might have gained. If you are out of touch with your body's inner voice, telling you what it needs, you might continue to eat out of the anxiety caused from the reality of weight gain. This hunger would be emotional hunger.

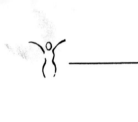

WEEKLY PATH WORK

1. Begin journaling about the definition of awareness and how it can be improved in your life.

2. What was **your** definition of awareness before you read Week 1?

3. Every night this week as you journal about your day in awareness, write down everything you ate during the day and the time of day it was. Now go back through your list and ask yourself each time were you responding to physical hunger, emotional hunger or spiritual hunger.

Also reflect upon whether or not you were in a place of awareness while you ate the food. Example: 10:00 muffin. Nervous about my job interview, so I ate from emotional hunger and I was not in awareness. I really wanted a cinnamon muffin but all I had in the kitchen was a bran muffin and that left me unsatisfied.

4. Every time you eat something, ask yourself how you feel. Be aware of how the sensation of food feels in your stomach. If you overeat, beyond satisfaction or to the point of being uncomfortably full, **do not panic!** All panicking will do is send you into a downward spiral of overeating. Be compassionate with yourself. Just say to yourself "that was great and I am now not going to eat again until I am physically hungry." This exercise puts you into a positive frame of mind. When we get angry at ourselves because we were not aware and we did overeat for whatever reason, we instantly go to the negative space of beating ourselves up. This will only set you up for the feeling of having failed, thus leading to more failure with compulsive overeating.

5. Every top of the hour during the day come to the place of awareness. No matter where you are or what you are doing, make a commitment to yourself that you are going to connect to yourself and be mindful throughout the day by checking in at 10:00, 11:00...the top of the hour. Journal about where you were with this exercise. Was this hourly check-in difficult? Easy? Why?

6. Every night during your journal time think about a different time in your life when you felt positive about your body. How do you feel about what was going on in your life at that time? What kind of clothes were you wearing? Where were you living? How old were you? Do you remember how it felt to move and to live within your body at the time?

7. Finish the sentence: I want to become more aware about my hungers and honor them appropriately because...

PATHWAY PROCESSING

This book is designed for you to stay in each section for a week in order to absorb the philosophy of that week's concept. Pick a night that symbolizes the beginning of the week for you, for instance Monday, then do the week through Sunday. Process what you connected to at the end of the week.

1. Did you journal every night for at least 20 minutes? If not how many nights were you able to write?

2. Were you able to check in every top of the hour and catch yourself being in a state of awareness?

3. Are you beginning to eat with awareness?

4. Note any thoughts or feelings you had surrounding any emotional or spiritual hungers you may have experienced throughout the week.

WEEK
2

THE PATHWAY TO HEALING:

BOUNDARIES

BOUNDARY (boun·`de·re)
indicating limits.

Compulsive overeaters often share a common problem. They have a lack of boundaries with people in their lives. People-pleasers want everyone to like them, so they inevitably over-extend themselves to others. When this occurs to the extent that it interferes with our own need for happiness, boundaries are collapsed and we are left feeling strained and even resentful. There may even be guilt over feeling resentment.

For example, if it makes you crazy that every time your partner or dear friend invites you out to eat they sit there and read the newspaper instead of talking to you, that is a boundary violation. Being dishonest about your personal limits or boundaries with the people in your life creates feelings of betrayal, anger, and defensiveness.

This only blows up in our faces as we become so resentful that we take it out on ourselves and overeat. My clients become aware of having no boundaries when they begin to work through the exercise of awareness. It is possible to be loving even as we begin to establish boundaries in our life.

I have found that as we become more compassionate with ourselves and establish the boundaries and personal space we need, we become more compassionate to those around us. When we are at peace with ourselves, we can more easily give to others in the ways that are meaningful.

New clients have had difficulty establishing their own boundaries between themselves and the outside world because so many emotions result from outside influences. We need to protect ourselves from others with strong boundaries.

Learning to stand up for yourself and honor your limits involves first noticing when you are being taken advantage of. You must learn to give yourself permission to have boundaries with the people in your life. In order to have good relationships with others, you must learn how to communicate your boundaries honestly.

The basic stages of boundary building

The process of developing a new relationship with food consists of: *Denial to awareness, awareness to commitment*, and finally *commitment to making the weight loss happen.*

When you stop denying and become aware of what you are eating and how much you are eating, this new awareness floats into every other area of your life. In the first few weeks of understanding this philosophy, new clients come to realize that they are the victims of the people closest to them, people who take full advantage of their over-generosity.

Boundaries, by definition, separate us from others. As we make our boundaries clear to others, we establish a certain amount of respect from the people in our lives. Only through this clarity can change take place.

There are some people who will come into your life and completely drain you of all your energy. I like to call these people 'boundary vampires'.

We all have someone or maybe a couple of people that just entered your thoughts as you read the previous description. Before you forget who they are, write them down. If you need a moment to think, take the time to write down the first 3 people that come into your mind:

1.

2.

3.

This exercise is important because we need to know our boundaries. Then we will be aware of who our boundary violators are.

A new client named "Mary" contacted me because she needed help losing the forty pounds she had gained during her two pregnancies. Her youngest child was 6. At first I wondered why Mary needed my help. Everything in her life seemed perfect. She and her husband owned a very successful company. When we first spoke Mary painted a picture of life being so perfect, filled with complete happiness. I knew that there must be an underlying reason Mary was using food to comfort herself.

After a few weeks of sessions she finally confided to me that all of their employees were her husband's relatives and most of them had the attitude that they were owed something and they did not work their 8 hour shifts. They did not hold regular schedules. It was also apparent that some of the family staff were skimming a sizable profit from the company

Mary, to her detriment, had no boundaries with these family members. She wanted desperately for them to love her. One of her biggest fears was that if she established boundaries with the family they would not love her and this would cause her to lose the love of her husband as well. So she said nothing to the boundary violators. Instead she would go home from work every night, exhausted and overworked, because she was doing the work of her employees. She would bathe her kids, put them to bed, and then begin to eat everything in sight. She was eating not from physical hunger, but from being frustrated at her husband's resentful family members, who were so blatantly taking advantage of her.

Mary began to realize that her weight problem was a direct result of her constant emotional hunger. A hunger caused from work and family related frustrations that she took out on food.

As she became more confident in establishing boundaries in her life she fired the employees who did not do their work and the other family members became model employees. As her boundaries became clearer her husband began to show her more respect. Mary lost weight and discovered more productive ways to deal with her stress. She began to feed her emotional hunger with craft classes at night because she was no longer doing the work of her staff. Her emotional hunger found a creative outlet.

We all know how to love other people in our life, now is the time to learn to love ourselves. The following exercise is a great journal assignment that can help you along this positive direction. Give this a lot of thought as you write about it during your evening journal time. Use your imagination. This represents you and your beauty, inside and out.

Boundary building exercise

Imagine that you are a beautiful garden. Think for moment about the flowers that would be planted there. Visualize what season it is and create your garden accordingly. Is it spring? Are there daffodils and tulips in your garden? Write about all the work it has taken to make your garden so abundant and special.

There is a velvety green lawn around your garden. There are footprints on it though, and there are holes in the flower beds where someone has carelessly cut out flowers. Who would do such a thing? Unfortunately, it's human nature for people to want to trample through a perfect lawn and pick the exquisite flowers that grow there. Often when there is no boundary, no fence, and we see beauty, we want to take a part of it home with us.

As you write about your garden think about building your fence. Be specific. How tall should it be? Approximately how close to your garden will it be placed? Close enough for people to lean over and still pick the flowers? The empowering part of this exercise is that we decide where we want to put this fence and how high it should be. How close should it be to your garden?

As you journal about this concept think about all the ways to build boundaries in your life with the people who are closest to you. As you get more comfortable establishing these new boundaries, you will have the self-confidence to begin establishing boundaries in every area in your life. As you do this more and more you will see the results in your relationship with food and compulsive overeating. You will no longer need to run to the refrigerator out of frustration from boundary vampires.

57

WEEKLY PATH WORK

1. Begin journaling about the definition of boundaries and about how you can improve the boundary system in your life.

2. What was your definition of boundaries before you read week 2?

3. One third of the people in your life will love you no matter what you do, one third of the people in your life will hate you no matter what you do, and one third of the people in your life won't care one way or the other, no matter what you do.

Draw three circles in your journal. In the first circle list the people in your life who love you no matter what you do. In the second circle list the people who hate you no matter what you do. In the third circle list the people who do not care one way or the other no matter what you do. Now, take a good look at these groups. Which circle do you want to share your precious time with?

4. Write about the boundary vampires in your life, past and present.

5. Imagine how your life will be affected once you have begun to establish clear boundaries. Describe how you think it will feel. Write about it.

6. Finish this sentence: I want to have boundaries with the people in my life because...

PATHWAY PROCESSING

1. Are you beginning to set boundaries with the people in your life?

2. Are you keeping your commitment to the evening journaling?

3. What other thoughts and feelings have come up this week? Feel free to release not only your lessons learned and positive reactions to the work, but any of your fears and doubts as well. Are you like Mary? Are you afraid to establish boundaries because you might lose the love of someone?

4. Remember, this is your unique healing process and there is no right or wrong way to connect to your true self.

WEEK
3

THE PATHWAY TO HEALING:

THE CHOICE TO SAY "NO"

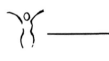

CHOICE (chois)
the right, power or opportunity to
choose an alternative.

NO (no)
not at all.

By learning to say "no" to others we are treating ourselves with respect and expecting others to respect us. The Buddhists believe in "dharma", meaning duty or purpose. We each have our own dharma. Focus on your own dharma by saying "no." In this week's assignment we will journal about our compulsive need to constantly say "yes" to everyone. This process will allow you to connect to your inner voice, a voice that may want (and certainly deserves) to say "no."

When the people in your life need something, are you the first person they call? Many compulsive overeaters share a common condition of desperately wanting everyone to love them. So the last thing we want to do is tell someone we are not available to do something for them.

When we spread ourselves too thin we begin to resent all the people that we are trying to please. Ultimately that sends us running, yet again, to the refrigerator to comfort our overworked nerves with food out of an enormous emotional hunger. When you let others take advantage of you by not saying "no" you are not honoring your limits. Having flexibility and being a "yes" person, are not the same thing. By trying to be everything to everyone we lose ourselves, we give ourselves away.

If you say "yes" when you really want to say "no" you are not communicating your limits honestly and you are setting yourself up for feelings of resentment, hostility, and even depression, all **emotional hungers.**

We can always keep a sense of balance in our lives by concentrating on the choice we have to say "no." This is hard for most people in the beginning but following the week of learning to build a fence around our beautiful garden will make it a lot easier. As we become more aware of the things in our life that cause us to eat from hungers other than physical hunger, the need to take care of ourselves first becomes clear.

It is *always* possible to choose the "no" word. Although we want to emphasize the positive and we fully intend to keep affirming it, we become acutely aware of the pain and suffering of learning to say "no" to those we really want to please. I admire the bravery and courage my clients have shown me as they have grown into their own strength. They learn to establish boundaries and say "no" to others. They realize that the more they give, the more is expected of them, and there is no break until they break internally from spreading themselves too thin.

We all know the woman who is very loving and supportive. She bakes for every bake sale, she volunteers for every food drive, she drives everyone else's kids around when the other parents are too busy or just won't. She is the woman who needs a haircut, needs new clothes right down to her bra and panties. This woman is also overweight and is probably overeating from extreme emotional hunger due to being in a state of resentment. She is always doing for others. Sound familiar? Are you her?

Are you like this? Do you find it difficult to say "no" to others for fear that you will not be liked? Are your fears so real that you attempt to get your needs met by taking care of others' needs first?

When someone like the woman mentioned above comes to me as a new client, she is so far removed from what her problem is, she cannot see how her inability to say "no" is ruining her life. It is as if she doesn't have her own life. Her life revolves around pleasing others.

As she begins to take stock in herself and trust in the strength of her own inner resources, only then can she heal her dysfunction with food.

The first step is for her to concentrate on putting herself first. She must be aware of her tendency to worry about the reactions of others when she is too busy to give of her time. Choosing to say "no" means taking such risks and confronting her fears about how others will react.

We must be willing to accept that some people may not react favorably to our attempt at self-preservation. In fact, some may not accept the fact that we are no longer their doormat.

As you discover who really matters in your life, the joy is overwhelming. You can experience the happiness that healthy relationships bring.

OUCH! I know it hurts. I have done this kind of work and believe me I was surprised to find out who my real friends were. It is often hard to take this reality lesson but the rewards far outweigh the initial difficulty. Self-deception can seem like a comfortable place to be, but it only produces apathy, discouragement, depression and ultimately an emotional or spiritual hunger we fill with food.

We all know how to say "yes" to everyone. In my practice I see my clients saying "yes" to everyone but themselves. Compulsive overeaters try to save the world because they are afraid to focus on saving themselves. We need to

67

care for ourselves as lovingly as we care for others. If we do not seek out time to take care of us, we are no good to our loved ones.

When we begin to say "no" to people we will ultimately re-kindle an interest in ourselves. With the new self-confidence you gain as a result of letting people know that you are not so available, your time becomes **YOURS.** You will begin to realize that every time you said "yes" to something you really did not want to do, you were not taking that precious time for yourself.

We are called on to say "no" everyday. **We** make the choice. Reclaim **your** power by saying **"no."** It is all about communicating to others what **you** really need.

WEEKLY PATH WORK

1. Begin journaling about your definition of what your choice to say "no" means and how it can improve your life.

2. What was your definition of the choice to say "no" before you read week 3?

3. Make a list of all the people in your life to whom you have a hard time saying "no."

4. Out of all the people in the list from assignment #3, who returns favors back to you?

5. Visualize yourself at a nice restaurant. You are with a friend and you are not particularly hungry. Imagine yourself saying "no" to ordering food when the waiter comes to take your orders. Picture yourself being totally ok with saying "no" to food and ordering a glass of water, an espresso or a glass of wine. That is all you order because that is all you want. How many times have you ordered food when you were not hungry because you felt uncomfortable about it or were intimidated by the restaurant staff?

6. Visualize yourself being put on the spot and asked to put together some type of event or help with a fund raiser. Imagine yourself feeling completely comfortable saying, "no, I just do not have the time to sacrifice right now."

7. Visualize saying "no" in any circumstance. For example: picking up people at airports, watering plants while others go on vacation, or helping someone move. Be strong in your command of the choice to say "no."

8. How much time do you spend each week devoted to activities for your own fulfillment? Be honest. How much time would you like to devote to yourself each week?

9. Finish this sentence; I want to have the choice to say "no" and feel good about that choice because...

PATHWAY PROCESSING

1. Are you beginning to have the confidence to say "no" to the people in your life?

2. How is the nighttime journaling going?

3. Are you gaining a sense of who you are, your true inner self and potential?

4. Are you realizing the power of being selfish with your time?

5. Are you beginning to understand how much you sacrifice for the happiness and convenience of others? Are you beginning to see a pattern with how you deal with your frustration and emotional eating?

WEEK
4

THE PATHWAY TO HEALING:

NEGATIVITY

NEGATIVITY (neg`a•tiv`i•ty)
lacking positive attributes.

As we become more aware of everything in our life from the food we are consuming to becoming aware of the simple daily events such as the drive to and from work, we begin to remove the layers of negativity surrounding our being. What is our pay-off for thinking negatively?

Many of us carry around a negative inner voice on a daily basis. This voice, taught to us either directly or indirectly, by parents, teachers, a coach or maybe a critical music teacher, stayed with us and we are so comfortable with the daily dialogue that it is hard to start a positive dialogue.

This is our work for the week. We need to acknowledge our negativity and find a positive way to release feelings of self-judgment.

Most of us have a strong habit of self criticism and self-judgment. This is called simply, being negative. Negative thinking keeps us from conquering compulsive overeating. When we are negative through self criticism, we instantly want to overeat. Stop focusing on the losing weight aspect of your ideal self. If you continue to focus on everything that might go wrong while you are trying to lose weight instead of focusing on what can go right, you will deny yourself healing in this area of your life.

The one thing we can count on in life is change. Learning to accept changes, especially if they are negative circumstances, helps us develop a stronger sense of self. As we become stronger in ourselves, we will stop running to the refrigerator in times of adversity or in moments of emotional insecurity. We need to accept the not so perfect situations in our life because guess what, things will change.

Negativity is damaging. It poisons our potential. Being negative leaves us emotionally fragile and conditioned for failure. Negative people create negative feelings in their environment, like the ripples in a pond from the toss of one pebble. Negative people tend to create an atmosphere, squashing other people's dreams because of their own issues (jealousy, fear, insecurity...) looking for reasons why recovery from compulsive overeating (or anything else for that matter) will not work for them or for you.

Unfortunately, we will always live in a world with such negativity. We must now ask ourselves to confront our own negative traps. Ask yourself, "am I one of the people contributing to the population of negative people?" If you are, how can you change? Surround yourself with the positive side of life. You have the right to positive forces in your world. Surround yourself with positive people, too. This is your choice.

It is so easy to have a day take a turn toward the negative. I personally have had days when promised checks do not show up in the mail, clients cancel at the last minute and I find out my dog has worms. But I have learned that, if negativity overwhelms me and I lose my sense of awareness, I will keep stepping out onto that negative pathway. When we are in a space of awareness and we have a day like this, we cannot let the negativity overwhelm us and send us running to the refrigerator.

I could easily bathe in my misery and disappointments after a day like this, and glue a big "L" for loser on my forehead.

Instead, I try and turn the negative into a positive. I find that due to cancellations, I have some time to work on my book. Due to lack of promised checks, I am forced to sit down and balance my checkbook, and due to the discovery of my dog's worm problem I am able to get medication for him and make him feel better.

My disappointments ultimately made me a more productive member of society that day and I was able to accomplish these important tasks without needing the comfort of food to temporarily feel better.

If we take a deep breath and focus on the positive side of life, we will be certain to attract positives. Of course, if we focus on the negative, then we begin to attract more of that into our lives. This is spiritual law.

I love the Bible scripture; "consider this my brethren when you encounter trials and tribulations. For the testing of your faith produces endurance..." In other words, that which does not kill you, makes you stronger. So consider it joyously when life gives you lemons, because you can make lemonade. I know it sounds cliche, but when a day that was supposed to be a certain way does not go as planned, try and see it in a new and positive light. Accept your challenges and comfort yourself with the thought that the testing of your patience by the universe only produces greater inner strength.

Lighten the negative impact by turning to the positive. As we allow each difficult experience to soften us and not instantly turn to the numbing comfort food, we will learn to attend to our emotional hunger in a positive way.

The basic source for any negative thought emerges because our expectations are not carried out. No one consciously decides to be negative. Ask yourself, "are the choices I am making in life leading me to exhibit negative or positive behavior? Does being negative or positive enhance my spiritual or emotional growth? How can I take small steps toward developing a more positive mind set?"

Now turn your attention toward helping yourself choose positive ways to deal with food. We cannot instantly make negativity leave all areas of our life but, if we stay aware and remember that we are larger than a negative feeling, we can at least begin to transcend the unwanted feeling.

Negative thoughts can lead us to feel anxious, isolated and out of control. You may recognize these as triggers to emotional eating. I have seen my clients crawl out of their negativity and lose weight as they discover new ways of thinking. They blossom by gaining strength and a new capacity for self-care. A negative experience or thought no longer leads them blindly toward food.

You can accentuate the positive without denying the unhappy aspects of your life. You will reclaim control over your life when you replace the negative thoughts that normally have control over you such as, " I will never lose weight" or "I will never feel good about my body."

Growing away from the habit of negative thinking allows us to move toward inner peace, a strong sense of self, a sense of joy and a feeling of control in your life. We are then able to bloom into our unique selves.

Take a moment to write out five disappointments in yesterday's plans that created negative thoughts and feelings:

1.

2.

3.

4.

5.

Now write five ways yesterday's disappointing schedule changes could have been viewed in a positive light:

1.

2.

3.

4.

5.

     Learning to plan for and deal with a tendency toward negativity will give you a stronger sense of self. The awareness of this tendency will gradually lead you to a more positive frame of mind.

     This week's assignments lend themselves to a positive mental preparation for negative emotions. Carry your journal around with you throughout the day in order to keep a record of events as they unfold. This is so you can measure your progress. When you feel the desire to eat, out of frustration or to comfort yourself because of emotional hunger; write instead.

WEEKLY PATH WORK

1. Begin journaling about the definition of negativity and how it can be improved in your life.

2. What was your definition of negativity and how has it changed since you read week 4?

3. Bearing in mind the importance of staying AWARE, remember to neutralize the tendency to react negatively with a positive response. When any negative situation comes along this week, focus on changing your first response, then the benefits of staying positive will be yours to enjoy. Keep a running list of the situations that arise and ask yourself how this negativity may have taken you on the downward spiral of compulsive eating.

4. We often get caught in the trap of assuming our negative emotions reflect the way things are in our life. Our perceptions do not always signify the reality. Make a list of three positive things going on in your life right now. You may want to include a new song you like, the adoration of your pet or even a great movie that inspired you.

5. Who inspires you? Why ? What positive qualities would you like to absorb from them? What is it about them that you like? Try to be specific.

6. Journal about your reactions throughout the day, whether they are positive or negative. Which ones escort you to the refrigerator when you are not physically hungry. Sit with your reactions, your thoughts, your feelings. Allow the truth to emerge. Perhaps confusion will come forth. That is ok too. But remember that constantly submerging yourself in negativity only serves to keep you stuck.

7. Finish this sentence: I want to release negativity from my life because...

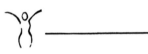

PATHWAY PROCESSING

1. Are you recognizing a tendency toward being negative? Is that tendency leading you down the path of compulsive overeating?

2. Has negativity kept you from your ideal weight?

3. Are you getting into a routine of nighttime journal writing?

4. Are you beginning to notice any new changes in your eating habits?

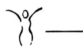

WEEK
5

THE PATHWAY TO HEALING:

A SENSE OF SELF

S E N S E (sense)
a perception or impression.

S E L F (self)
the individuality or nature of a person.
the ego.

Sense-of-self healing involves befriending your body at the weight you are right now. Your work will only be defeated if you keep resisting acceptance of yourself at your present weight. Accept yourself along the journey to your desired weight, not when you have attained some goal on a scale. We unconsciously believe that reaching our goals of weight loss will not only give our lives meaning but deliver happiness and protect us from pain and suffering. The belief that a sudden strong sense of self will suddenly emerge if you reach your ideal weight or size is a false belief. We must separate fantasy from reality. No matter how much weight you lose, you must cultivate a sense of self before you can live in your body comfortably. In fact, I have found that when my clients begin to accept their bodies as is, they begin to lose weight more easily. This is because they are coming from a place of calm and self-love. I understand how difficult it is to accept yourself **now.** Remember, it is a gradual process. Think of it as a self-acceptance project.

When you spend time this week journaling about rediscovering and healing your sense of self, one of the things that you must do is ask yourself, "when did I lose that part of myself, or did I ever have a strong sense of self?" The power of having a strong sense of self is the most important determining factor in reaching our goals of:

1). Ideal weight
2). Freedom from food obsession.

Abusing food with compulsive overeating interferes with your ability to appreciate your unique self. In order to change your relationship with yourself, you must change how you see and feel about yourself. Until you begin to love yourself as you are today, you cannot change in a meaningful and lasting way.

Many of us are in the habit of comparing our self with others' physical appearances. Do you have that person in your life who has the body you always wished for or even the lifestyle you always wanted? Comparing yourself with anyone else makes it nearly impossible for you to develop self-knowledge and ultimately self-worth. We need to feel connected to ourselves, period. Constantly comparing yourself to others is a waste of time and energy. It sets up the cycle of feeling good when you are around people you rate favorably against and feeling down when you are around those whom you feel somehow inferior to...of course it would be impossible to go through life without ever comparing ourselves to others. How we become unique individuals depends on how we look at ourselves in relation to others, right? We want to break the mold, and we can. Otherwise, we will not recognize the inner strength we have hidden from ourselves. It will not magically appear if we are busy living through someone else, or wishing that we could.

Some clients have shared with me that the best time of their lives was when they were at a certain weight and everything else in their life was so "perfect." They seem to think that they had their strongest sense of self then. But why did they regain the weight and hold onto the fantasy of that particular time? Furthermore, why do they feel it is their fault, their innate weakness, for not maintaining that "perfect weight"? It is time to focus on the **now.**

When we build our sense of self foundation on sand, the first storm will cause it to collapse. The possibility of a long-standing foundation is gone. We are left empty and lost.

It is impossible to love yourself and have a sense of self if you do not approve of who you are at the weight you are right now. To believe that your self-worth depends on the shape of your body or a certain magical number on the scale is counter productive. Your sense of self must come from your love for yourself in this moment. Growing into a strong sense of self is a task one must do alone. No one else can do it for you.

A major step toward acceptance of your sense of self involves releasing the negative body image and making room for a positive self image. In doing so, you are able to release a great deal of self-hate and self-disgust that was wrapped up in your previously negative sense of self.

The last time I vacationed in Mexico, I was captivated by a group of women who were at the pool of my resort. There were five of them and all were at least 60 to 100 pounds overweight. These women were gorgeous. Everyday they came out to the pool in new ensembles: gold lamé swimsuits, matching sandals complete with gold lamé bows, straw purses filled with manicuring kits, the latest fashion magazines and decorative water bottles. These women held the whole poolside's attention. They were all so sensual, so genuinely beautiful. What they had in common and what they had that most women at the pool did not have was a strong sense of self. They believed in their beauty and took good care in adorning themselves at their present size. Their inner light was so powerful that the women seemed to glow.

As shown by this group of women, it is very important to dress in clothes that make you feel good about your body at the size you are right now. You might have to put some energy into an extra trip or two to the mall, but the clothes are readily available. It will be well worth the effort. Do not convince yourself to wait until you are a perfect size 14, 12, 10, 8. We decide what goes *in* our body and we need to be in charge of what we put *on* our body as well.

When I was living at the City of Hope Cancer Treatment Center, while my husband was going through cancer treatment, I discovered that the patients there all had one thing in common: a strong sense of self. These people were physically weak, bald and puffy from steroids, but they were all painfully aware of their chances of survival and their commitment to fighting for life. I was aware of their complete acceptance of who they were as individuals. They made an effort to enjoy their life moment to moment and seemed content to be themselves. They did not waste time comparing themselves to others.

A common pothole we all fall into is comparing ourselves with others. Maybe one of the reasons we feel inclined to do this is our fear of discovering who we really are.

We all have days when our sense of self is the size of a dime, when we are uncomfortable in our own skin. We tend to emotionally distance our mind from our body size. Often, we think we are a lot bigger than we really are. However, as you learn to accept yourself and love yourself today at the weight you are now, then an inner peace begins to transform you . Even other people will notice your new attitude about yourself, and the glow that such a transformation will bring. This is a very slow process, but will stay with you and make you aware of the beauty in your own body.

I often recall one client in particular who began to realize her beauty. She was so overwhelmed with her new love of self that she wrote me to share her feelings:

"...something weird happened the other day, a major milestone in my healing. I was looking at my large body in the mirror after my shower and instead of turning away from the mirror, I looked. I noticed my breasts and realized they really aren't ugly at all.

For years I hated them because my nipples were placed low on my breasts. But I noticed them the other day and this doesn't make them ugly. They're very full. They certainly are not wrinkly or saggy or gross. I had a plan for 5 years from now that I would save $3000.00 to have surgery done to place the nipple higher. I was determined to do this until last week.

When I first saw my breasts and didn't hate them I thought that this feeling would not last, that I would see them again in the mirror the next day and see how horrible they were. But that never happened. I saw them in the mirror the next day and they didn't look horrible. I'm not going so far as to say that my breasts are great or anything, but I've stopped hating them so much. I wasn't even working on a strong sense of self, it just happened. I told my husband about it and he said, 'your breasts were never ugly, it was all in your head.' All I keep thinking about is how much I have healed..."

* * *

Part of having a strong sense of self involves releasing our concern about how others may view us. Since our society defines our achievements based upon what others think, we have fallen into the trap of believing other opinions about us. So many people are unhappy with their bodies, regardless of what the scale says. One of the important goals of the **journey to the shape of you,** is to inspire you to reclaim your sense of self through the journal exercises. The best motivator to lose weight is not fitting into a certain size of clothing, it is recovering your sense of self.

I don't mean to imply that we should walk around in a state of euphoria all of the time. But we do need to reach a place of contentment within and about our own being. The opposite of unhappiness is happiness. But with body image, the opposite of unhappiness should be contentment with our body. Only then will we find inner peace.

Now is the time to get to know yourself. Instead of focusing on the outside, focus on the inside. Get to know yourself apart from the weight issues. There is no one else like you on earth.

WEEKLY PATH WORK

1. Begin journaling about the definition of "sense of self" and how it can be improved in your life.

2. What was your definition of "sense of self" before you read week 5?

3. Describe a time in your life when you had the strongest sense of self? What did you weigh? How long a period of time was it? Did the feeling go away when you gained weight?

4. Write about where you were with your sense of self and body image a year ago today? What kind of clothes were you adorning yourself in?

5. Whom do you know or who have you observed who has a strong sense of self? What could you do to apply some of their self image into your life?

6. Journal about any situation where you have compared your self to someone who you felt was physically better than you. How did this comparison make you feel? Did it send you running to the refrigerator? Now think about a child that you love, a child that is very close to your heart. If that child shared with you this same story of judging him/herself against someone else, what advice would you give them? Would you not want that child to see the beauty in themselves?

7. Write a page introducing yourself to a room full of strangers. Pretend that in the audience there is a potential lover, employer, or neighbor. Sell yourself to them, the self you are at this moment. Read back what you would say. Does it surprise you?

8. Finish this sentence: I want to have a strong sense of self because....

PATHWAY PROCESSING

1. How are your evening journal assignments going?

2. Are you becoming aware of your own beauty?

3. Are you finding it difficult to accept yourself at the weight you are right now? Why is that?

4. What thoughts and feelings emerge? Challenge yourself to self-acceptance.

5. How might you learn to further your belief in yourself?

WEEK
6

THE PATHWAY TO HEALING:
THE BELIEF THAT I DESERVE

D E S E R V E (di zurv`)
to be worthy of.

What do you believe you deserve? Kindness and nurturing? Or do you have a distorted belief, one that suggests you do not deserve, because of your present weight? It is very important to believe that deserving is not about your size, it is about your attitude. We are going to spend this week exploring this concept.

The belief that "I deserve..." is reminding ourselves that we deserve. Then we can begin to believe it and start claiming that belief into our life.

The people I work with share similar stories. Over and over, the details are different but the basic feeling is the same. They feel that they do not deserve to be an active participant in life if they are at an unfavorable weight.

I often hear statements like: "...I do not deserve to go to my best friend's wedding because I'm fat and have nothing to wear. I do not deserve to go to the nicer department store and purchase my vacation clothes because I am fat, so I'll go to a discount store and buy cheap, poorly fitting, fake fabric clothes to wear because I do not deserve to wear clothes that feel good at this weight..."

I find that when my clients first come to me they spend about 75% of their time obsessed with food, hating their bodies and wanting to change their feelings about both. When we feel worthy of deserving, it increases our chances for happiness.

There is a high cost to feeling that you do not deserve. Often times, by believing that we do not deserve, it causes us to stay stuck at a low point or worse yet, drop even lower.

When we neglect our needs it is because we lack the essential sense of deserving. We must accept that we have the right, even the responsibility to be good to ourselves. Believing in the fact that you deserve affirms the healthiest message you can deliver to your conscious and subconscious mind: "I deserve to take care of all of my needs."

Every person has the potential to believe that they deserve. But it is a choice. It is up to you to **choose** to feel deserving. We are the star of our own life story, a journey that takes place from birth until death. As we travel the pathway of life it is certain that we will encounter pain, loneliness, vulnerability, and self-doubt. We will know the frustration of life's limitations and we will also discover love, happiness and inner wisdom.

My clients have taught me that it is not simply what happened to them that shaped who they are. It is what happened within them that made the difference. When they felt undeserving of belonging at a particular place because of their size, instead they would stay home and eat. The goal is to enjoy eating as a part of a full life instead of eating to deal with an empty one. Getting over this hurdle is hard and it requires telling yourself that **you deserve.**

If you continue to give yourself to this healing process, I can assure you that your journey will be more fruitful than you could ever imagine.

How can you learn to reach this level of confidence, feeling that you deserve? How can you get to a space of accepting your body at the weight it is now and feeling strong enough to go out and celebrate life?

Tell yourself, "I deserve." Many clients think about the process of losing weight and then feel unworthy of a thin person's life. What it usually boils down to is that they are not ready for the thin side of life because they do not believe they deserve it. Your goal is to begin reminding yourself gently, you are ready for the best life has to offer on all levels because you do indeed deserve.

WEEKLY PATH WORK

1. Begin journaling about the definition of "I deserve" and how it can be improved in your life.

2. What was your definition of "I deserve" before you read Week 6?

3. Start a list of I deserves.in your journal.
Example: I deserve to get a facial. I deserve to buy some pretty new sheets for my bed...list at least 10 things during your evening journal time.

4. Do you remember a time in your life when you felt more deserving? What was your body like then, compared to now?

5. Do you deserve to treat yourself with compassion?

6. Are you deserving of a thin person's life? Does that scare you?

7. Finish this sentence: I want to feel like I deserve because...

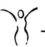

PATHWAY PROCESSING

1. How do you feel about yourself in general after reading Week 6? Do you think you deserve to be your ideal weight? If not, then what is blocking you?

2. Have you been carrying around your journal during the day? Are you finding the writing a replacement for emotional eating?

3. Make a list of the things you feel you deserve, things that are realistically attainable in the next 4 weeks.

WEEK
7

THE PATHWAY TO HEALING:

BLAME

B L A M E (blam)
to hold responsible.

The easiest way to keep from growing and conquering compulsive overeating is to stay in a space of blame. This week will be about healing the many reasons we find to blame. We can break the blame mentality when we heal our relationship with food and body image.

We cannot explore our feelings of blame until we acknowledge that they exist. Many of us have learned to numb our feelings with food. Perhaps we do not even realize that we live in a state of blame. If we internalize blame and do not acknowledge that we do so, we will continue to eat out of resentment.

The dreaded days of self-loathing can begin with blaming a pair of panty hose not fitting quite right or a new pair of jeans shrinking on the first wash, thus making you feel fat. These are not reasons to blame or punish ourselves with self-loathing, are they?

We all have frustrations and personal failures regardless of weight. Dieting leads people to insist on instant gratification. The minute they have reached their ideal weight, boom!!! The weight comes back on. Why? They go back to their old eating habits. But guess what? They blame everything and everyone for the weight gain.. The diet did not fail you . You failed yourself by not healing the wounds that cause you to compulsively overeat and numb yourself with food. Through the diet you changed nothing. In order to change we must be aware of our strengths and weaknesses, while simultaneously letting go of that tendency to blame.

It is easy to be a victim and blame others for your weight problem and poor body image. Blame is a form of self-pity, and self-pity is negative. Negative feelings send us running to the refrigerator. So knowing this, realize the futility of the blame. It only harms **YOU**.

Blaming others or situations allows you to maintain a false self-image. It buys you time until you can come up with better targets of blame or more excuses for not healing compulsive overeating. Blame will allow you to live with your own imperfections and still feel ".vindicated" about staying overweight. We can blame our weight gain or overeating on everything from vacation, stress, hurt feelings, childhood, pregnancy, menopause...relying on blame is an act of desperation. These things should not be blamed on your body. Nor should you blame your less than ideal body on these things. We must break away from this cycle.

Blaming all the sources of your eating problem keeps you stuck. When you take responsibility for a problem you take control by becoming empowered. We create our own destiny. Keep in mind it takes time to learn how to blame yourself for being a size you are not happy with and remember it takes effort to be kind to yourself too, about as much effort as it takes to be mean to yourself. So why not spend the energy on kindness?

When we blame our compulsion to overeat, or our weight gain on anything but ourselves, we are left powerless and the ideal of growth seems impossible . It is counter productive to blame. We need to accept responsibility. Before you take back your power, you must first be able to recognize that you do have a problem with blaming. This involves catching yourself in the act.

Once we stop blaming others, events, or simple daily challenges (like the weather) as being responsible for our relationship with food and our dissatisfaction with our body size, we can heal these wounds and move on.

Many people blame their weight for every failure or disappointment that comes their way. When we encounter a failure or disappointment in life it can cause us to feel fat instantly. We need to stop relating those failures and disappointments to our size. In a recent session with a client, I learned that every time she spent time with her mother, she felt fat the next day. This feeling made her turn to ice cream for comfort. She blamed her mother for causing her to turn to food. Then she blamed herself for feeling powerless over food. She blamed her mother for causing her to feel so fat and weak.

Was it really her mother's fault or did she give her power through blaming? Do you find yourself falling into the blame game?

WEEKLY PATH WORK

1. Begin journaling about the definition of blame and how it can be improved in you life.

2. What was your definition of blame before you read Week 7?

3. Recall a memory of blame that sent you rushing to comfort yourself with food.

4. Make 3 columns. The first column is for anyone you blame. The second column is for the reasons you blame him or her. The third column is for how this blame affects you.

5. What actions can you take to decrease the amount of energy you spend on blaming yourself, others, or circumstances in your life?

6. In what ways has blame kept you from having a positive self-image?

7. What situations cause you to quickly react to blame?

8. Finish this sentence: I want to stop blaming others, situations and things out of my control for my compulsive overeating because....

PATHWAY PROCESSING

1. Were you consistent with the evening journal assignments? Have you accepted this journaling as a permanent part of your recovery from compulsive overeating?

2. Are you beginning to comfort yourself with writing in your journal instead of turning to food to feed your emotional or spiritual hungers?

3. Is it hard to be honest with yourself in admitting a tendency to blame?

4. Has blame kept you from recovery from compulsive overeating?

EPILOGUE

JOURNEY TO
THE SHAPE OF YOU

The seven steps in this book are not a pathway with a clear beginning and end. They are an ongoing opportunity for you to change your relationship with food and enjoy your new and improved self. It is scary to succeed. Embrace your success but do not forget the work it took to get there.

When you lose weight you may find that people will treat you differently. Be aware of all those well meaning people who will loudly acknowledge your weight loss to a room full of strangers. Please do not run to the refrigerator to deal with the anxiety that such an event may provoke.

Remember all of the things you did right. Remember these last seven weeks and all of the things you learned about yourself. It is extremely important to validate yourself this way for two reasons:

1. Your success has nothing to do with luck.

2. Hard work does pay off.

The underlying theme here is: It is not about the food. We need to live within awareness. We need to have boundaries with the people in our lives. We need to be comfortable enough with ourselves to say "no, I really do not have the time." We need to remain positive. Do not dwell in the ever abundant negativity. We need to have a strong sense of self at the weight we are right now. We need to believe that we deserve. We need to learn not to blame.

We cannot go through life afraid of change. Personal growth comes from the result of facing changes directly and dealing with them successfully. Do not be afraid of change, embrace it.

The only roadblock to change is fear. And remember, **the opposite of fear is trust...**

You will maintain your success because you worked through issues common to compulsive overeaters. Keep reminding yourself of the basics.

If you apply one or two lessons from this book to your life it will make a significant difference in your relationship with food and body image. Lasting change with food is a learning curve. The patterns that keep us stuck in the vicious cycle of compulsive overeating can be changed as long as we trust that we have the power to make those changes.

GOOD LUCK!

PART 2

JOURNAL TO
THE SHAPE OF YOU
WORKBOOK

Journey to The Shape of You Journal Workbook was created to help people learn through the exercise of journaling, that it is not what you are eating, it is what is eating at you. It is possible to lose weight without a diet. Diets simply do not work. All a diet does is put a Band-Aid on a wound. Writing is a form of therapy, through writing in this journal you will travel to the real reason you choose to comfort yourself with food. You will finally heal that wound once and for all.

In our society, we want instant gratification. That is why so many people will turn to a diet boasting weight loss results of 20 pounds in 6 weeks. Unfortunately, it will usually be followed by a regaining 25 pound in 10 weeks.

Healing yourself from the inside out takes longer. The results of conquering compulsive overeating through self-awareness are forever. This book is designed to help you raise your awareness and re-connect to your inner voice of physical hunger.

As compulsive overeaters we use food to numb ourselves. The way we heal our relationship with food is by first healing deprivation which has created an obsession with food.

If I were to say; "you can never have another banana for the rest of your life," you instantly crave a banana. Immediately you will become obsessed with bananas. Banana pie, banana bread, ice cream etc. Because the sense of impending deprivation would make you think you are hungry for a particular food. You might not even like bananas, but the thought of never being able to have one again somehow makes you suddenly crave one.

This kind of deprivation is where diets fail people. It has been said if you need to gain weight, go on a diet.

Next, we must learn to listen to our body, not our mind, with regard to food cravings. Often our first response in encountering this step involves fear. "What if I crave chocolate?" **We must remember that the opposite of fear is trust.** In working this step with the journal we begin to recognize where we go wrong in our relationship with food. All we need to do is, eat when we are physically hungry, eat what we are hungry for, and stop when we are satisfied. Practically applying these steps in your daily life is a challenge.

In the journal you will begin to recognize when you are physically hungry. You will learn as you write to differentiate between physical, emotional and spiritual hungers. When you trust your body and honor your physical hunger, you well discover what it truly means to be satisfied with food, as opposed to that uncomfortable feeling of eating beyond satisfaction. **The only reward to eating beyond satisfaction is weight gain.**

WHY JOURNAL?

As we begin the process of healing our relationship with food, we begin to uncover all the reasons that lead us to compulsively overeat. In the journal you will initiate the healing of your relationship with food by uncovering the real reasons you used food to numb yourself in the first place.

Journaling brings forth an inner guidance for life's problems and allows individuals to connect to their own wisdom. During the process of re-connecting to physical hunger, you begin to release the many layers which cover the underlying problems that have caused you to be compulsive with food.

If you have previously kept a journal, consider this journal a renewed devotion to healing your dysfunction with food. In the journal, allow yourself to become self-centered, by this I mean more centered in self.

As you become more grounded in yourself through daily journaling, the pages will lead you to a deeper understanding. You will begin to see how you became disconnected to your inner wisdom and began to comfort yourself with food.

The journal writing experience creates powerful insights about ourselves. Writing on a daily basis in the journal enables us to identify and ultimately "feed" our emotional and spiritual hungers.

There is no right or wrong way to journal. To make a commitment to lose weight and work on the reasons you have used food to numb your pain, fill up your loneliness or even release anxiety is difficult. Journal writing will increase self-understanding and self- esteem.

We all want self love and inner peace. We all need to have a positive self image and a strong sense of self. Through journal writing we can explore the inner truth without shame. The page is not concerned with logic, only healing. What we are writing becomes a channel to our growth.

GETTING STARTED

The initial decision to start a journal is yours. In today's fast paced society we get caught up in fulfilling so many external obligations that we end up neglecting our own needs. The result is a feeling of resentment and a profound sense of emptiness that usually sends us running to the refrigerator for comfort. It is a vicious cycle that leaves us feeling empty and unhappy.

I recommend journal writing to become a part of your everyday life. The best time to journal is right before you go to bed. Make it a special time and plan on at least 20 minutes before you go to sleep. Curl up in that favorite chair or get into your bed and surround yourself with your pillows. This should be an exercise of self-nurturing so make the most out of the experience by getting totally comfortable and relaxed.

Begin by journaling about your day and reflect on your experiences with food. Did you eat when you were not hungry? Why was that? What triggered the eating?

In a few weeks go back and reflect on the pages. Is there a pattern to any dysfunctional experiences with food? Maybe there is a daily challenge to be aware of. Understand and explore these feelings.

The point is to get to know yourself better and recognize the stumbling blocks that keep you from your ideal weight.

If there is an evening where you are not inspired to write, read and reflect on the statements in the journal pages. Let that guide you with your evening writing. Draining your brain in the journal from the day's events will be a release you will begin to look forward to.

There are no rules. If you feel inclined to journal at other times during the day then go right ahead. I love to journal in the afternoons at my local coffee house.

This is your journal experience. Make the most of it. Welcome to your Journey to the Shape of You.

REMEMBER:

Often, the thing which we resist the most in life
is the very thing keeping us from our dreams.
What do you resist?

JOURNALING

is a pathway to a strong sense of self.
On a scale of 1-10 where would you measure
your sense of self?

SPENDING
time in solitude with your journal
is a self-nurturing activity.
How much time did you spend
with your journal this week?

Did you spend your day in total
AWARENESS?

It is not what you are eating,
it is what is eating at you
that keeps you from your ideal weight.
What is eating at you?

1/3 of the people in your life will love you
no matter what you do,
1/3 of the people in your life will hate you
no matter what you do,
and 1/3 of the people in your life
will not care about you one way or the other
no matter what you do.
Who are the beloved 1/3 in your life?

What is your ideal body size?

The one thing we can count on in life is change. Does change cause you to be emotionally hungry?

Journal about the boundaries you have
with the people in your life.
Do you have boundaries with
the people in your life?

How comfortable are you with
your choice to tell people "no"?
Does it cause you to feel resentful,
anxious or guilty when you agree to do something
you were too uncomfortable to say "no" to?
Do these uncomfortable feelings cause you
to run to the refrigerator?

What makes you feel negative?

Do you have a strong sense of self?
Do you compare yourself to others?
Be honest.

Every day make a list of
10 great things you deserve!!!

Journal about blame.
Who do you blame?
What do you blame?

Writing is a form of therapy.
Through writing, we explore our
inner truth without shame.

Through journaling, learn to get in touch
with the silence within yourself.
That is where all of your answers are.

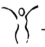

SHOOT FOR THE MOON!
Even if you miss you will land among the stars.

The only reward for eating when
you are not physically hungry
is weight gain or maintaining a weight
you're not happy with.

ABOUT THE AUTHOR

Marian Willingham lives in Northern California with her two dogs, Libby and Max. As a Personal Eating Coach her practice includes clients in the United States, Canada and Europe. In her spare time, Marian enjoys restoring vintage homes and going to flea markets.

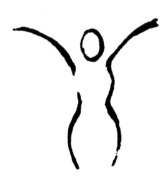

If you would like to order the companion
Journal Workbook
please send this order form
and a check or money order for $12.00
(CA residents add 87¢ sales tax)
which includes S&H to:
The Shape of You
Journal Workbook Order
241 N. Washington St.
Cloverdale, CA 95425

Name: _____

Address: _____

City: _____State:_____Zip:_____

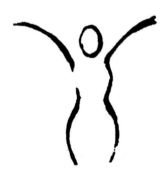

THE SHAPE OF YOU

To order a free catalog
or for more information on
working with a Personal Eating Coach
visit our website at
www.theshapeofyou.com
or call
707-894-0655

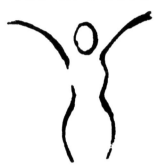

If you would like to order the
quarterly newsletter "Positive Images"
please send a check or money order for $12 to:
The Shape of You
241 N. Washington St.
Cloverdale, CA 95425
Please make checks payable to
The Shape of You